# LOWER CHOLESTEROL NATURALLY

## How to Reduce High Cholesterol with Natural Remedies

# James Edwards

# TABLE OF CONTENTS


INTRODUCTION

CHAPTER ONE

What You Need to Know About Cholesterol

CHAPTER TWO

The Importance of Natural Cholesterol Reduction

CHAPTER THREE

Diet and Nutrition for Naturally Lowering Cholesterol

CHAPTER FOUR

Natural Cholesterol Lowering Lifestyle Changes

CHAPTER FIVE

Natural Cholesterol-Lowering Supplements and Remedies

CHAPTER SIX

The Mind-Body Connection for Controlling Cholesterol

CHAPTER SEVEN

Monitoring Results and Remaining Committed

CONCLUSION

# INTRODUCTION

The pursuit of good health has become a top priority for many people in today's busy world. The fast-paced world we live in frequently leaves little room for the care and attention our bodies require, and the consequences of this neglect can be subtle or severe. High cholesterol, a silent but formidable foe, infiltrates our veins, increasing the risk of heart disease, one of the leading causes of death worldwide.

But, in the midst of this seemingly insurmountable challenge, there is an empowering truth: you have the power to take control of your health and, as a result, naturally lower your cholesterol levels. We embark on an illuminating journey into the complexities of cholesterol control in this book, 'Lower Cholesterol Naturally: How to Reduce High Cholesterol with Natural Remedies,' revealing a wealth of scientifically-backed, natural strategies that can help you regain command of your cardiovascular well-being.

The pages that follow will guide you through the confusion of cholesterol reduction, providing not only a thorough comprehension of the subject but also a wide range of practical techniques and lifestyle changes that could help lower cholesterol. You will learn how to make use of nature's healing power, making informed choices that help lower your cholesterol levels without the use of excessive medications or invasive procedures.

'Lower Cholesterol Naturally: How to Reduce High Cholesterol with Natural Remedies' is more than just a guide; it is your companion on the road to a healthier heart. By the end of the book, you'll have the knowledge and tools you need to make long-lasting, positive changes in your life. Your path to lower cholesterol and better health starts here.

# CHAPTER ONE

## What You Need to Know About Cholesterol

It's important to understand cholesterol if you want to live a healthier life and avoid heart disease. Cholesterol is a complicated topic that's viewed as a negative consequence, but it is necessary for many bodily functions. In this chapter, we'll look at what cholesterol is, the different types of cholesterol, how it affects your health, and why it's so important to control.

**Understanding Good Cholesterol and Bad Cholesterol**

Cholesterol is a lustrous, fat-like substance found in all of your cells. It is required for the formation of cell membranes, the production of hormones, and the digestion of fats. Lipoproteins, which carry cholesterol in your blood, are classified into two types:

1. Low-Density Lipoprotein (LDL): Also known as "bad" cholesterol, LDL transports cholesterol from the liver to cells throughout the body. Too much LDL cholesterol in your bloodstream can cause plaque buildup in your arteries, a condition known as atherosclerosis. This accumulation narrows the arteries, reducing blood flow and raising the risk of heart disease.

2. High-Density Lipoprotein (HDL): HDL is commonly referred to as "good" cholesterol because it aids in the removal of LDL cholesterol from the bloodstream. Excess LDL cholesterol is transported by HDL back to the liver, where it is processed and eliminated from the body. It means that a high HDL cholesterol level is important to reduce the risk of heart disease.

## Your Health and Cholesterol

The levels of both HDL and LDL Cholesterol in your body are highly significant to your overall health, especially your cardiovascular health. You are more likely to develop heart disease if your LDL cholesterol levels are too high and your HDL levels are too low. This is how it works:

## Atherosclerosis

Atherosclerosis is a disease condition in which plaques form in the arteries of the blood vessels. This plaque is made up of cholesterol, fatty acids, calcium, and other substances. Plaque hardens and narrows the arteries over time, reducing blood flow. This can result in a variety of cardiovascular issues, including:

- Coronary Artery Disease (CAD): Narrowing of the coronary arteries, which supply blood to the heart, can cause chest pain (angina) or a heart attack.

- Stroke: A stroke can occur if plaque builds up in the arteries supplying blood to the brain.

## Cholesterol and Cardiovascular Disease

High LDL cholesterol levels are a major risk factor for cardiovascular disease. When LDL cholesterol oxidizes, it can cause artery inflammation. The inflammatory response of your body can result in the formation of blood clots, which can block blood flow and cause heart attacks or strokes.

## The Function of Triglycerides

Triglycerides are another type of fat found in your blood, in addition to LDL and HDL cholesterol. Triglyceride levels are also associated with an increased risk of heart disease, particularly when combined with high LDL cholesterol.

**Keypoints of Cholesterol Control**

Given the importance of cholesterol in your health, it is important to control it properly. The following are important points to consider in the quest to control cholesterol:

1. Know Your Numbers: Have your cholesterol levels checked on a regular basis. This will assist you in understanding your current situation and setting goals for improvement.

2. Lifestyle Influences Cholesterol Levels: Among the most important factors influencing cholesterol levels are lifestyle choices. A healthy diet, regular exercise, and not smoking can all help to keep cholesterol levels in check.

3. Dietary Changes: Cutting back on saturated and trans fats, increasing fiber, and choosing healthier fats can help lower LDL cholesterol and boost HDL levels.

4. Medication: Medication may be required in some cases to control cholesterol levels. Your healthcare provider can advise you on whether this is the best option for you.

Understanding cholesterol is the first step toward naturally lowering it and protecting your heart health. You can control your cholesterol levels and reduce your risk of heart disease by making informed choices and taking proactive steps. This chapter has established what cholesterol is and why it is important. We will look at practical steps and strategies for naturally lowering your cholesterol and promoting a healthier heart in the following chapters.

# CHAPTER TWO

## The Importance of Natural Cholesterol Reduction

In our hasty society, it's all too tempting to put our health on the back burner in favor of convenience and rapid satisfaction. To address health issues such as high cholesterol, we frequently rely on quick solutions and pharmaceutical interventions. While drugs can be useful, they also have side effects and long-term implications. In this chapter, we'll look at the strong reasons to favor natural cholesterol reduction.

### 1. Long-term Wellness and Health

Natural cholesterol reduction is a path toward long-term health and wellness. Unlike drugs, which may provide quick results, the natural approach to cholesterol control strives to build long-term habits that will benefit you for the rest of your life. This is a worthwhile journey because it covers more than just reducing cholesterol but improves the general health of an individual.

### 2. Lessening of Side Effects

While pharmaceutical cholesterol-lowering medicines are beneficial, they frequently have negative effects. These might range from minor symptoms such as headaches and stomach problems to more serious difficulties such as muscle pain and liver problems. By using natural approaches, you lower your chances of experiencing these negative side effects, allowing your body to repair and balance itself without intervention from synthetic ingredients.

## 3. Improved Quality of Life

Lowering cholesterol naturally can improve one's quality of life. You'll most likely have more energy, a better mood, and less stress. When you take control of your health through lifestyle changes, you receive a sense of control and empowerment, which improves your overall well-being.

## 4. Cost-cutting measures

Pharmaceutical treatments can be costly, especially when used over an extended period of time. Natural approaches, on the other hand, are frequently less expensive. Investing in a heart-healthy diet, getting regular exercise, and controlling stress with relaxation techniques are all reasonably inexpensive options that can offer considerable health advantages.

## 5. Improved Heart Health

Natural cholesterol-lowering approaches not only cut cholesterol levels but also improve overall heart health. They help to reduce blood pressure, and inflammation, and improve blood vessel function. This all-encompassing approach reduces the risk of heart disease and its complications.

## 6. Long-Term Results

Although medications provide temporary relief, they do not treat the underlying reasons for high cholesterol. Natural methods, on the other hand, seek to address the underlying causes of increased cholesterol levels. You have a better chance of attaining long-term results if you make durable adjustments to your food and lifestyle.

7. Less reliance on medications

You may be able to lessen your dependency on cholesterol-lowering drugs if you lower your cholesterol naturally. This is especially useful for people who are concerned about the potential side effects and long-term repercussions of prescription medications. Working toward natural solutions gives you the ability to take charge of your health.


8. Individualized Approach

Natural cholesterol control enables a customizable approach that is suited to your specific needs and preferences. You can try out various diets, exercise routines, and stress-reduction approaches to see what works best for you. Because it is tailored to your specific lifestyle and goals, this personalized approach can produce more long-term effects.


9. Healthy Aging

Lowering cholesterol naturally is an investment in your future, not just the present. Maintaining optimum cholesterol levels becomes increasingly important as you age. Adopting a natural approach to cholesterol management will help you live a healthier life later in life by lowering your risk of chronic diseases and improving your quality of life.


Finally, the significance of naturally lowering cholesterol cannot be overstated. It is a journey toward long-term health, fewer side effects, a higher quality of life, cost savings, improved heart health, long-term results, less medication dependency, a personalized approach, and healthier aging. This chapter has laid the groundwork for comprehending the numerous advantages of using a natural approach to cholesterol management. The chapters that follow will go into greater detail about the specific strategies and lifestyle changes that will help you achieve your cholesterol goals naturally.

# CHAPTER THREE

# Diet and Nutrition for Naturally Lowering Cholesterol

One of the most potent and long-lasting ways to naturally lower cholesterol levels is to maintain a healthy diet. You can significantly lower your risk of heart disease and enhance your general health by making wise food choices. This chapter will discuss the fundamentals of a cholesterol-friendly diet and give you useful advice and meal suggestions to assist you in reaching your objectives.

## Knowledge of Cholesterol

It's crucial to comprehend the various types of cholesterol before moving on to dietary strategies:

1. Low-Density Lipoprotein (LDL): Frequently referred to as 'bad' cholesterol, elevated levels of LDL can raise the risk of atherosclerosis and heart disease.

2. High-Density Lipoprotein (HDL): Also known as 'good' cholesterol, HDL aids in the removal of excess cholesterol from the bloodstream, lowering the risk of plaque buildup in the arteries.

3. Total Cholesterol: The sum of your LDL and HDL cholesterol levels.

4. Triglycerides: A type of blood fat that, when elevated, can contribute to heart disease.

**A Cardiovascular-Healthy Diet**

1. Consume Plant-Based Foods: A plant-based diet can be extremely effective in naturally lowering cholesterol. Include a variety of fruits and vegetables, whole grains, legumes, and nuts in your daily diet. These foods are high in fiber, antioxidants, and nutrients that aid in LDL cholesterol reduction.

2. Choose Healthy Fats: Choose unsaturated fats such as those found in olive oil, and avocados, and fatty fish such as salmon and mackerel. These fats can raise HDL cholesterol levels while decreasing LDL cholesterol.

3. Limit Saturated Fats: Saturated fats are commonly found in red meat, full-fat dairy products, and processed foods. These fats have the potential to raise LDL cholesterol levels.

4. Avoid Trans Fats: Trans fats, which are commonly found in partially hydrogenated oils in processed and fried foods, can raise LDL cholesterol while decreasing HDL cholesterol. Avoid products that contain trans fats by reading food labels.

5. Increase Soluble Fiber: Soluble fiber-rich foods like oats, beans, and fruits like apples can help lower LDL cholesterol levels by binding to cholesterol and removing it from the body.

6. Omega-3 Fatty Acids: Include omega-3 fatty acid sources in your diet, such as walnuts, flaxseeds, and fatty fish. Omega-3 fatty acids can lower triglycerides and lower the risk of heart disease.

**Meal Plan Example**

Breakfast:

- Oatmeal with fresh berries and ground flaxseeds on top.

- A glass of orange juice that has just been naturally squeezed out from a fresh orange fruit.

- Herbal tea or black coffee (no cream or sugar added).

Lunch:

- A sizable mixed green salad with chickpeas, tomatoes, cucumbers, and an olive oil vinaigrette dressing.

- A portion of brown rice or quinoa made from whole grains.

- A few almonds that are unsalted.

Snack:

- A fruit serving, like an apple or a banana.

- Natural yogurt dollop.

Dinner:

- Salmon with a lemon and dill sauce baked or grilled.

- Steamed carrots and broccoli.

- Either brown rice or quinoa.

Dessert when necessary:

- A tiny square of dark chocolate that contains at least 70% cocoa.

Keep in mind to sip water frequently throughout the day. In addition to supporting your body's natural ability to manage cholesterol, staying hydrated is essential for overall health.

**Here are Important Points to Note:**

- Examine food labels to find hidden trans and saturated fats.

- Use canola, avocado, and other heart-healthy oils when preparing food.

- Instead of using too much salt to flavor your food, use herbs and spices.

- Portion control is essential because even healthy foods if consumed in excess, can cause weight gain.

You can lower your cholesterol naturally and lower your risk of heart disease by changing your diet and leading a heart-healthy lifestyle. Prior to making any significant dietary changes, always seek the advice of a medical professional or a registered dietitian, especially if you are currently taking medication or have a medical condition. They can offer you individualized advice to assist you in effectively and safely lowering your cholesterol.

# CHAPTER FOUR

# Natural Cholesterol Lowering Lifestyle Changes

Making lifestyle changes is one of the most important steps in your natural cholesterol-lowering journey. These modifications not only lower your cholesterol but also improve your overall health and well-being. Adopting a heart-healthy lifestyle can significantly reduce your risk of heart disease and allow you to live a longer, healthier life.

## Understanding the Relationship Between Cholesterol and Lifestyle

Before diving into the practical changes you can make, it's critical to understand the connection between your lifestyle and your cholesterol levels. Cholesterol is a fatty substance produced by your liver and found in your food. They are made up of two types including low-density lipoprotein-carrying (LDL) cholesterol and high-density lipoprotein-carrying (HDL) cholesterol. LDL cholesterol is commonly referred to as "bad" cholesterol because it can accumulate in your arteries, increasing your risk of heart disease. HDL, on the other hand, is referred to as "good" cholesterol because it assists in the removal of excess cholesterol from the bloodstream.

Lifestyle factors are important in controlling cholesterol. Unhealthy habits like poor diet, lack of exercise, and smoking can raise LDL cholesterol while decreasing HDL cholesterol. Making positive lifestyle changes, on the other hand, can reverse these effects, increasing HDL cholesterol while decreasing LDL cholesterol.

**The Nutritional Advantage**

Your diet is one of the most important factors in cholesterol control. The following dietary changes can help you naturally lower your cholesterol levels:

1. Select fats that are heart-healthy:

Healthy alternatives like the monounsaturated and polyunsaturated fats found in olive oil, avocados, nuts, and seeds can be used in place of trans and saturated fats.

2. Boost Soluble Fiber

Oats, beans, fruits, and vegetables are examples of foods high in soluble fiber that can lower LDL cholesterol levels.

3. Increase Your Omega-3 Fatty Acid Intake:

To increase HDL cholesterol and lower triglycerides, add nuts, mackerel, and other fatty fish to your diet.

4. Reduce Cholesterol Consumption:

Limit your intake of foods high in cholesterol, such as organ meats, egg yolks, and full-fat dairy.

5. Mind Your Portion Size:

To control calorie intake and maintain a healthy weight, pay attention to portion sizes.

## The Value of Consistent Exercise

Another crucial element of a heart-healthy lifestyle is physical activity. Exercise can improve your cardiovascular health by lowering LDL cholesterol and raising HDL cholesterol. Aim for at least 150 minutes per week of moderate-intensity aerobic exercise or 75 minutes per week of vigorous-intensity aerobic exercise, along with at least two days per week of strength training. Swimming, cycling, and brisk walking are all great ways to increase your heart rate and strengthen your cardiovascular system.

## Quitting smoking

Smoking raises cholesterol levels and is a significant risk factor for heart disease. One of the most important lifestyle changes you can make for the health of your heart is to stop smoking if you currently do so. To improve your chances of success, look for assistance from smoking cessation programs, medications, and a strong support network.

## Controlling Stress

Chronic stress can lead to unhealthy lifestyle decisions like poor eating habits and inactivity, which can then have an impact on your cholesterol levels. Discovering stress-reduction techniques that work, like meditation, yoga, mindfulness, or relaxing hobbies, can enhance your general health and cholesterol profile.

## Getting to and Keeping a Healthy Weight

Keeping a healthy weight is essential for controlling cholesterol. If weight loss is necessary, it can significantly affect your cholesterol levels. The secret to achieving and maintaining a healthy weight is to combine a proper diet with regular exercise.

**Regular Examinations and Supervision**

Finally, it's crucial to regularly assess your progress. This entails setting up routine checkups with your doctor to monitor your cholesterol levels and general health. It also entails understanding your genetic predisposition to high cholesterol and remaining informed about your family history. Based on this information, your healthcare provider can help you customize lifestyle changes and, if required, suggest medications to effectively manage your cholesterol.

Making these lifestyle changes a part of your daily routine can have a significant impact on your cholesterol levels and overall cardiovascular health. Remember that the journey to naturally lower cholesterol is a marathon, not a sprint. Small, sustainable lifestyle changes can have a big impact in the long run, lowering your risk of heart disease and allowing you to live a longer, healthier life.

# CHAPTER FIVE

# Natural Cholesterol-Lowering Supplements and Remedies

In the pursuit of reducing cholesterol naturally, it becomes important for us to consider natural supplements and remedies. While a healthy diet and regular exercise are important components of controlling cholesterol, these additional measures can supplement your efforts and help you meet your cholesterol-lowering targets. In this chapter, we'll look at some natural supplements and remedies that have shown promise in lowering cholesterol and improving heart health.

## 1. Sterols and Stanols from Plants:

Plant sterols and stanols are naturally occurring compounds found in a variety of plant-based foods, including nuts, seeds, and vegetables. They work by preventing dietary cholesterol absorption in the intestines. Certain margarine and spreads fortified with plant sterols or stanols can help lower LDL (low-density lipoprotein) cholesterol. For a noticeable effect, you must incorporate these into your daily diet.

## 2. Omega-3 Fatty Acids:

Omega-3 fatty acids, which are found in fatty fish (such as salmon, mackerel, and sardines), flaxseeds, chia seeds, and walnuts, have been shown to benefit heart health. They have the ability to lower triglycerides, decrease inflammation, and promote healthier blood vessels. If dietary sources are limited, aim for at least two servings of fatty fish per week, or consider high-quality fish oil supplements.

3. Garlic:

Garlic is a naturally occurring plant substance that has been used in the past for medicinal purposes. According to some studies, garlic may help lower total cholesterol and, in particular, LDL cholesterol. If you don't like the taste of garlic, you can use garlic supplements or add it to your cooking.

4. CoQ10 (Coenzyme Q10):

CoQ10 is an antioxidant produced by the body that aids in the production of energy in cells. Some cholesterol-lowering medications, such as statins, can deplete CoQ10 levels. Taking CoQ10 supplements may help to reduce statin side effects and improve heart health.

5. Red Yeast Rice:

Red yeast rice is a traditional Chinese medicine made by fermenting rice with yeast. It contains compounds that are similar to those found in statin medications and has been shown to reduce LDL cholesterol. However, before taking red yeast rice supplements, consult with a healthcare professional because their effectiveness varies and they may interact with other medications.

6. Green Tea:

Catechins, which are powerful antioxidants found in green tea, may help lower LDL cholesterol levels and improve overall cardiovascular health. Regularly drinking green tea or taking green tea extract supplements can help you manage your cholesterol.

7. Psyllium Husk:

Psyllium husk, a soluble fiber derived from the seeds of the Plantago ovata plant, has been shown to help lower LDL cholesterol levels. It prevents cholesterol absorption by binding to it in the digestive tract. For a fiber boost, mix psyllium husk into water or incorporate it into recipes.

8. Vitamin B3 (Niacin):

Niacin is a B vitamin that can increase HDL cholesterol while decreasing LDL cholesterol. However, due to the possibility of side effects, it should only be used under medical supervision. Niacin supplementation should be discussed with a healthcare provider because high doses can cause flushing and liver problems.

9. Berberine:

Berberine is a plant compound that can be found in a variety of plants, including goldenseal and barberry. According to research, it may help lower cholesterol levels and improve overall heart health. Berberine, like other supplements, should be used after consulting with a healthcare professional.

10. Curcumin and turmeric:

Curcumin, the active compound in turmeric, is well-known for its anti-inflammatory and antioxidant properties. According to some studies, curcumin may help lower LDL cholesterol levels and reduce the risk of heart disease. Including turmeric in your cooking or taking curcumin supplements can help.

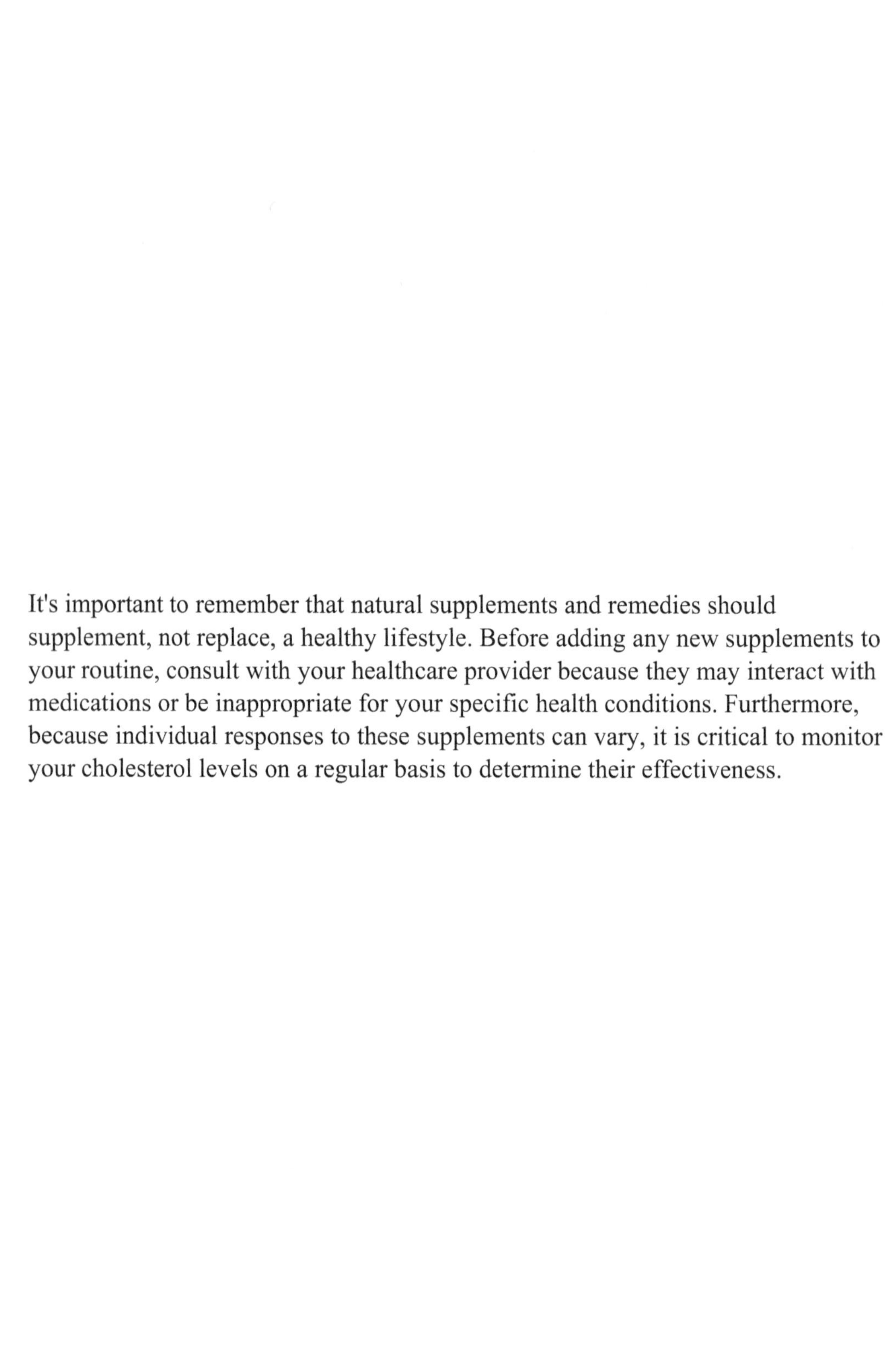

It's important to remember that natural supplements and remedies should supplement, not replace, a healthy lifestyle. Before adding any new supplements to your routine, consult with your healthcare provider because they may interact with medications or be inappropriate for your specific health conditions. Furthermore, because individual responses to these supplements can vary, it is critical to monitor your cholesterol levels on a regular basis to determine their effectiveness.

# CHAPTER SIX

# The Mind-Body Connection for Controlling Cholesterol

The relationship between the mind and body is very important for maintaining overall health, which includes controlling cholesterol levels. This chapter will examine the profound effects that your thoughts, feelings, and level of stress may have on your cholesterol profile as well as how you can naturally lower your cholesterol by utilizing the power of the mind-body connection.

## Stress and Cholesterol

Stress has ingrained itself into contemporary life of this days. The hormone cortisol, also known as the "stress hormone," is released by our bodies when we are under stress. While cortisol is crucial in fight-or-flight situations, prolonged stress can cause this hormone to be produced in excess, which can lead to a number of health problems, including high cholesterol levels.

Stress can cause people to make unhealthy lifestyle decisions, including those related to smoking, poor eating habits, and inactivity — all of which are known risk factors for high cholesterol. The composition of your blood's cholesterol can also be directly impacted by stress, with levels of low-density lipoprotein (LDL) cholesterol or "bad" cholesterol, which can clog your arteries, rising.

## Conscious Eating

The relationship between the mind and body starts with how you eat. Being present in the present moment while you eat is encouraged by the practice of mindful eating. You can better tune in to your body's hunger and fullness cues by paying close attention to the flavors, textures, and smells of your food. This can assist you in limiting your intake and selecting healthier foods.

You're less likely to reach for comfort foods high in sugar and saturated fats when you eat mindfully. You'll instead gain a stronger understanding of your body's nutritional requirements, which will make it simpler for you to select heart-healthy foods high in fiber, antioxidants, and healthy fats.

## Meditation and Relaxation

By lowering stress and the production of cortisol, relaxation techniques like meditation and yoga can have a significant impact on your cholesterol levels. You can improve your cardiovascular health by meditating to clear your mind and reduce the feeling of worry. Daily mindfulness meditation for just a few minutes can make a big difference.

You can also enhance your mind-body connection and manage stress by practicing yoga, tai chi, and deep breathing techniques. These exercises promote relaxation, increase heart rate variability, and may eventually have a positive impact on your cholesterol profile.

## The Feeling Heart

Another crucial element of the mind-body connection is your emotional health. Your health, including your cholesterol levels, can be negatively impacted by negative emotions like anger, depression, and anxiety. Chronically unhappy feelings can influence blood lipid levels, inflammation, and poor lifestyle decisions.

It is important for your general well-being to develop emotional resilience and to ask for assistance when necessary. You can support the health of your heart by navigating emotional challenges with the aid of supportive relationships, counseling, and stress-reduction techniques.

## The Influence of Vision

A strong tool for achieving your health goals is visualization. You can inspire yourself to make better decisions by visualizing your body operating at its peak, with clean and clear arteries. When combined with other stress-reduction techniques, visualization can be especially powerful.

## Your Own Phrase to Lower Cholesterol

Consider creating a personal mantra or affirmation to help you manage your cholesterol by utilizing the mind-body connection. A straightforward statement like "I am in control of my cholesterol levels" can keep you inspired and committed to your wellness objectives. Regularly repeat your mantra, especially when you feel stressed or tempted.

In conclusion, the mind-body connection is crucial to your efforts to naturally lower cholesterol. Your journey to better heart health can be assisted by stress reduction, mindful eating, relaxation techniques, emotional well-being, visualization, and personal mantras. You can control your cholesterol levels more holistically and live a healthier, happier life by being aware of and fostering this mind-body connection.

# CHAPTER SEVEN

## Monitoring Results and Remaining Committed

Naturally lowering your cholesterol is a noble goal, and as you set out on this journey, it's important to have a plan in place to monitor your success and keep up your commitment. This chapter will walk you through the significance of keeping an eye on your cholesterol levels, give you tips for staying on track, and give you advice on how to stay motivated as you work toward better heart health.

**The Need to Monitor Cholesterol Levels**

Monitoring your cholesterol levels is a critical step in your pursuit to lower cholesterol naturally. It accomplishes several things:

1. Monitor Development

You can determine how successful your efforts are at lowering cholesterol naturally by routinely checking your cholesterol levels. It enables you to determine which lifestyle changes have a positive impact and which one that needs to be altered.

2. Maintain Your Knowledge of Your Cholesterol Level

Cholesterol levels can fluctuate over time due to a variety of factors, so keeping track of your numbers ensures you are aware of any potential issues early on. Knowledge is an extremely effective tool for gaining control of your health.

3. Inspiration

Seeing visible changes in your cholesterol levels can be a powerful motivator. When you see the positive results of your lifestyle changes, it strengthens your resolve to continue making healthy choices.

**How to Monitor Your Progress**

Follow these steps to effectively monitor your cholesterol levels:

1. Speak with Your Healthcare Provider

It is critical to consult your healthcare provider before making any changes to your cholesterol-lowering plan. They can advise you on the best tests and intervals for monitoring your cholesterol.

2. Arrange for regular blood tests

Schedule regular blood tests to measure your cholesterol levels, as directed by your healthcare provider. A lipid profile, which measures total cholesterol, LDL (low-density lipoprotein), HDL (high-density lipoprotein), and triglycerides, is typically included in these tests.

## 3. Keep a Cholesterol Journal

Maintain a journal in which you can record your test results and track your progress over time. Include the date and results of each test, as well as any relevant lifestyle changes.

## 4. Establish Realistic Goals

Set attainable cholesterol goals in consultation with your healthcare provider. The goal that you should set should be a measurable cogent goal. For example, you could aim to lower your LDL cholesterol by 20% in six months.

## 5. Make Use of Technology

Use smartphone apps or online tools to keep track of your cholesterol levels and lifestyle changes. These tools frequently provide visual representations of your progress, which helps you stay motivated.

## Maintaining Focus

Maintaining a commitment to naturally lowering cholesterol can be difficult, but it is critical for your long-term health. The following are important clues that you should observe to maintain your focus:

## 1. Continue Your Education

Continue to educate yourself on the most recent cholesterol and heart health research and information. Understanding the motivations behind your actions can help you stay committed.

## 2. Establish a Support System

Share your goals with your friends and family and solicit their help. Having a network of people who encourage and motivate you can make a big difference in your level of commitment.

## 3. Rejoice in Small Victories

As you go along in the process, you should endeavor to celebrate small wins. These achievements, whether it's a decrease in LDL cholesterol or sticking to a healthy eating plan, should be recognized and rewarded.

## 4. Review Your Objectives

Review your cholesterol-lowering goals on a regular basis and make adjustments as needed. If you've accomplished one goal, set a new one to keep your motivation high.

## 5. Visualize Your Achievement

Visualize the advantages of naturally lowering your cholesterol. Imagine a healthier, more active lifestyle, and use this vision to keep your commitment going.

## 6. Seek Professional Help

If your commitment wanes or you face difficulties, consider seeking the assistance of a registered dietitian, nutritionist, or healthcare provider. They can offer advice, support, and new perspectives.

Remember that lowering cholesterol naturally is a gradual process with potential setbacks. Stay patient and persistent, and you will reap the benefits of your commitment to better heart health in time.

# CONCLUSION

Finally, lowering cholesterol naturally is a journey that is laden with blessing and hope. Making small but significant changes to your lifestyle, diet, and general health can have a significant impact on your cholesterol levels, as we've discussed throughout this book. You've unlocked the potential to lower your risk of heart disease, improve your vitality, and improve the quality of your life by being proactive about your health and relying on nature's cures.

Keep in mind that improving your cholesterol requires more than just giving up certain foods or following a brief fad diet. It involves developing enduring habits that support your body and safeguard your heart. We've provided helpful advice, delectable recipes, and insightful commentary throughout this book to assist you in achieving your cholesterol-lowering objectives naturally.

The journey does not, however, end here. It carries over into your day-to-day decisions and dedication to a heart-healthy lifestyle. You'll not only lower your cholesterol as you put the information and strategies from this book into action, but you'll also feel better and more alive. Your future self will appreciate your commitment, and your heart will thank you.

So use the knowledge you've gained, accept the natural remedies provided, and start down the path to a healthier, cholesterol-balanced life. I hope this book will be your inspiration and a guide to living a more active, happy, and heart-healthy life in addition to naturally lowering your cholesterol. With each heart-healthy decision you make, the future becomes brighter. You have the power to protect your heart from the menace of 'bad' cholesterol.